Kunekune Pigs for Starters:

Full Guide on Kunekune Pigs, Tips, Their Care Including Breeding Matters and Health Issues and More

By

Laetitia S. Cormier

Copyright@2023

TABLE OF CONTENTS

CHAPTER 1

INTRODUCTION

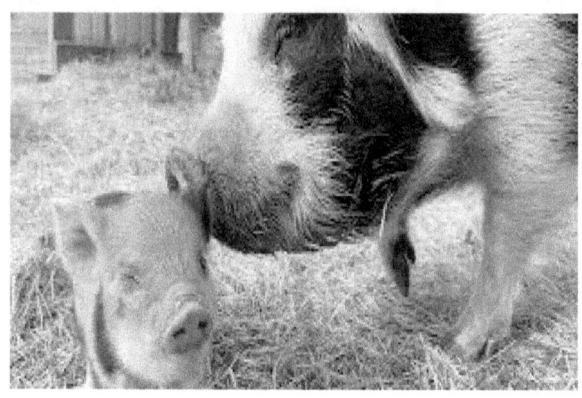

The domesticated pigs (that is, Sus scrofa domesticus) kunekune is tiny and shaggy. Kunekunes have a strong connection to the Māori, an indigenous population from island New Zealand. The Māori word kunekune translates to "fat and round".

Kunekune pigs graze, unlike most domestic pigs. They thrive on grass alone.

Kunekune pigs are gregarious and run to meet their caregivers in the morning.

Body Description

Kunekune pigs are little domestic pigs. These pigs have silky, coarse, or curly hair and come in cream, black, ginger, brown, as well as white. They have solid or speckled coats. Their hair also gets warmer or just thicker with the seasons and sheds in warmer months. Many kunekune hogs have fleshy "piri piri" wattles on their faces. They have semi-lopped ears and curled tails.

Size

Kunekunes are smaller than most domestic pigs. Adults can reach a height of four feet (1.2 meters) length and twenty-four inches sixty centimeters) tall. Female kunekune pigs (called "sows") weigh 120-200 lbs (54-90 kilograms), while males (called "boars") can reach 200-300 pounds.

Natural Habitat

Pigs, domestic counterparts of wild boars, may flourish in many settings. The kunekune breed's origin is uncertain, however it resembles domestic pigs from Asia, South America, as well as the Polynesian Islands. Modern kunekune pigs may have originated from whalers who brought them to New Zealand during the 19th century and traded among the Māori people.

Communication

Kunekune pigs communicate by vocalization, body language, and scent markers. A happy, low-pitched grunt usually indicates pig relaxation. They additionally emit this noise when meeting. Pigs show tension or anxiety with high-pitched calls. These pigs express their feelings by waving their tails and ears.

Kunekune pigs typically live 15-20 years.

CHAPTER 2

TIPS FOR RAISING KUNEKUNE PIGS

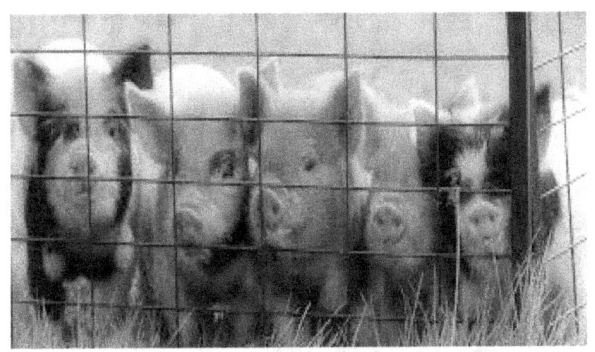

Here are top real implications or secrets:

Kune Kunes don't root. They graze grass. Like cows, they munch the backyard grass all day without turning it into mud (perhaps because their hair protects them from the sun?).

They grow to be heavy despite looking like a 40-pound dog. They are quite smart.

They enjoy being petted, particularly ear scratching and belly rubs. They love having their ears rubbed, then lean into the contact, and finally flop onto their backs and lift their hooves for a belly rub! Like a dog. Absolutely hilarious. They enjoy it so much they lay there afterwards to suck it up.

Their gentleness surpasses that of dogs, making them ideal pets for children. I often wear flip-flops around within the backyard while they keep going. Sometimes, my kids gently feed them from their palms without nipping!

Escape only occurs when they run low on food or water. I installed a wire fence in the pig's pen since they were escaping, but I found they required fresh water. Their escape attempts have ceased. The electric barrier has stopped working, as I recently discovered. Unsure how long it's broken!

They eat grass in summer without extra food! In winter, they can easily be fed alfalfa pellets, tiny pig feed, and table scraps.

They poop like giant animals while being small. I alternate between the backyard as well as the pig enclosure (side field), and following a few days in one place, their toilet area is covered. This product dissolves into the grass with rainwater, making it lush in May. However, in winter, when the grass isn't growing and April showers haven't occurred, the area is unusable. (They devote 1/3 – 1/2 of a full acre for their restroom.)

They're crazy fast. Luckily, by 1 year old, piglets' skin is thick enough for ticks to cling.

CHAPTER 3

FACTS REGARDING KUNEKUNE PIGS

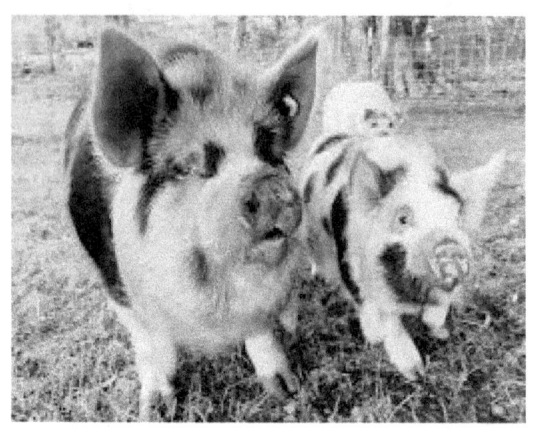

The Average Size of a Kunekune Pig

Female pigs, known as gilts or sows, normally weigh between 100 and 175 pounds when fully grown, while male pigs, known as boars or barrows, can reach weights of 200 to over 250 pounds. They can grow to a maximum of 450 lbs and 2.5 feet in length.

Despite their diminutive stature, kunekunes make for sturdy pets.

For What Purpose Are Kunekune Pigs Bred?

Kunekune pigs are reared for more than just their meat. They are wonderful companion pets because to their kind natures and placid demeanor, but their full size should be taken into account. Once again, their little stature belies their hefty weight.

Should One Get a Kunekune Pig as a Pet?

Due in large part to their mild demeanor, kunekunes are highly recommended as pets, especially for those who have never had a pig before. Unlike many other breeds, this one actually enjoys interacting with humans. Kunekune pigs are known for their playful, social, and goofy nature toward their human companions. They resemble huge canines.

Kunekunes are exceptionally bright and responsive to training, but their brilliance can easily be channeled toward harmful ends if it isn't challenged frequently enough. Training, intellectual stimulation, attention, and consistent socialization all contribute to their flourishing.

Before taking home a kunekune, it's crucial that you verify on any regulations, legislation, or restrictions in your area. You should also check that your home and yard can accommodate a 200-pound or larger animal.

While pigs as pets might be entertaining to have around the house, kunekunes need regular access to the outside so they can graze. In the same way that cats and dogs enjoy both the indoors and outdoors, so do these pigs. This favourite should be carefully put into notice.

Can Kunekune Pigs Be Consumed?

Kunekune pigs take longer to reach maturity than other breeds. Meat from these animals is crimson in color and has a lot of flavor, although it is enveloped by an outermost layer of fat. Its coating of fat seals in the breed's signature flavor and results in exceptionally delicate, juicy meat.

Also, kunekunes create a lot of delicious lard for cooking.

CHAPTER 4

KUNEKUNE PIGS CARE: HOUSE & FENCING, DIETS, AND THEIR TEMPERAMENT

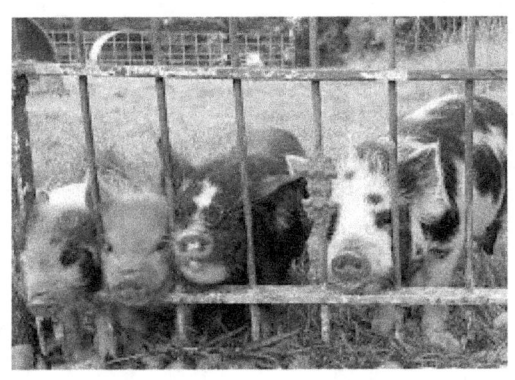

Kunekune Pigs and Homes

Little maintenance makes the kunekune pig the easiest to care for. Simple shelter and fence are enough to satisfy these pigs. Your gentle breed won't be harmful, but they can act out without mental stimulation and companionship.

Can Kunekune Swine Be Pastured?

Kunekune pigs are huge grass eaters and will eat almost just grass. Shelter against the elements is needed in the pasture. As long as the opposite side blocks winds, 3-sided buildings perform well.

The constructions must fit all your pigs comfortably. In chilly weather, they cuddle, but in summer, they prefer their space. Pigs require mud holes to cool down in heat.

Did you know that pigs sunburn easily?

Mud acts as sunblock, so they crawl in it to wrap themselves up. Since pigs sweat via their snout, they need other cooling methods. Mudholes are great for body temperature regulation.

Kunekune Pig Fencing

Kunekune pigs can be fenced like sheep or goats. Electric fence can be utilized, but young pigs should learn to respect boundaries. Not everyone needs electric fencing.

Kunekune Pigs: Destructive?

Unlike other pig breeds, kunekune pigs are less destructive. They eat without digging, preserving pastures.

Due to their submissiveness, they don't like challenging fences.

Due to their intelligence, they may intentionally act out when they feel neglected, whether by a lack of intellectual stimulation or your attention. They don't act destructively with sufficient care, excitement, and attention.

Winter Kunekune Pigs

Kunekune pigs are cold-hardy and rarely need heat. New or newborn piglets require extra heat to stay safe and warm. Your sow's winter piglets need a warming lamp.

Please install heat lamps or heat sources to prevent barn or structure fires. No heat lights should touch animals, beds, structures, or just any other thing that might heat up or cause a fire.

Pigs instinctively curl up for body heat, keeping them warm in winter. Extra hay as well as bedding are excellent for one pig in winter.

Pigs seek physical touch with other pigs even if they don't form vast herds. Having a single kunekune pig can make them lonely.

Kunekune Pig Feeding

Kunekune pigs can graze with no rooting of things to find food since their snouts point up. They graze heavily. Depending on grass amount and quality, kune diets may require grains. Depending on climate, winter supplementation is necessary.

Kunekunes like various fruits and vegetables like other pigs.

CHAPTER 5

KUNEKUNE PIGS: BREEDING MATTERS, THEIR HEALTH AND CONCLUSION

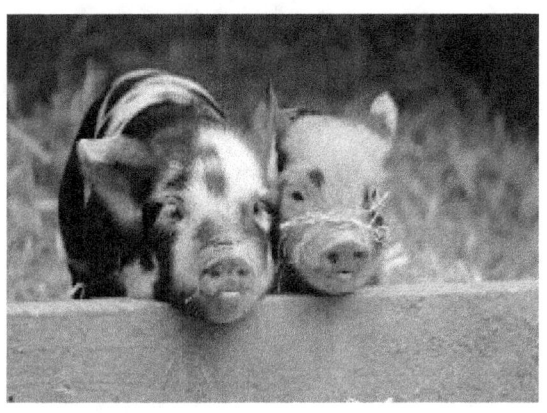

Breeding Kunekune Pigs

Kunekune boars can breed at 8 months but are not fully fertile until a year. Secondary traits appear about 18 months.

A sow's heat phase lasts 8–48 hours as well as repeats every 18–22 days until she falls pregnant. About 116 days pass during pregnancy. A sow should go to a birth pen a week before delivery.

Kunekune sows are excellent moms and raise piglets easily. A typical litter has 6-8 piglets. Because sows abort or reabsorb fetuses, a tiny litter of single or double piglets is unusual.

Kunekune boars can be infertile. Boar fertility varies by season. Extreme heat and cold reduce their fecundity.

Kunekune sows have unique infertility. Infection, hormonal disorders, or obesity can harm sows' reproductive tracts, causing infertility.

Hormone therapy can last a few months. If it fails, some farmers may cull or sell her as a pet.

Health Issues in Kunekune Pigs?

Kunekune pigs can get diarrhea. Dietary changes or bacterial illnesses can cause this. Young pigs can die from rotaviruses and E. coli infections.

Kunekune pigs get bronchitis, pneumonia, as well as nasal infections. Lungworms can cause coughing, as well as respiratory illnesses.

Piglets might be unviable due to congenital defects. One issue is being born with no an anus. Heritable health issues like scrotal or just umbilical hernias prevent pig breeding.

Sows can give birth early or abort due to toxoplasmosis, parvovirus, and leptospirosis. Because leptospirosis is zoonotic, stillborn piglets have to be treated carefully to prevent human transmission.

Kunekunes get lice and mange. Mange causes crusty spots, poor thrift, and slow growth.

One Last Thought

Kunekune pigs are smart, amiable, gentle, and lively. They love kids and people, unlike many other breeds. They make great pets and farm animals because of this.

THE END.